HOW TO BUILD A HEALTHY LIFE

Your roadmap to a better and longer life.

Dr. Elizabeth Hunter

Table contents

Chapter 1

A healthy diet often contains nutrient-dense foods from all of the main food categories, including lean proteins, whole grains, healthy fats, and fruits and vegetables of different colors. Healthy eating habits also include substituting items that include trans fats, added salt, and sugar with more healthy ones.

Following a nutritious diet has several advantages, including growing strong bones, protecting the heart, avoiding illness, and increasing mood.

Heart health

According to the Centers for Disease Control and Prevention (CDC)Trusted Source, heart disease is the top cause of mortality for people in the United States.

The American Heart Association (AHA)Trusted Source claims that approximately half of U.S.

individuals live with some sort of cardiovascular disease.

High blood pressure, or hypertension, is an increasing problem in the U.S. The disorder may lead to a heart attack, cardiac failure, and a stroke. It may be able to avoid up to 80% of premature heart disease and stroke diagnoses through lifestyle modifications, such as increased physical activity and a nutritious diet. The meals individuals consume may decrease their blood pressure and help maintain their heart health.

The DASH diet, or the Dietary Approaches to Stop Hypertension diet, contains lots of heart-healthy foods. The program recommends:

- eating lots of veggies, fruits, and whole grains
- selecting fat-free or reduced fat dairy products, fish, poultry, legumes, nuts, and vegetable oils

- minimizing saturated and trans fat consumption, such as rich meats and full-fat dairy products\slimiting beverages and meals that include added sugars
- reducing sodium intake to fewer than 2,300 milligrams per day — preferably 1,500 mg daily — and boosting consumption of potassium, magnesium, and calcium

High-fiber diets are also vital for keeping the heart healthy.

The AHA believes that dietary fiber helps improve blood cholesterol and decreases the risk of heart disease, stroke, obesity, and type 2 diabetes. The medical profession has long recognized the relationship between trans fats and heart-related disorders, such as coronary heart disease.

Limiting certain kinds of fats may also benefit heart health. For instance, reducing trans fats decreases the levels of low-density lipoprotein (LDL) cholesterol. This form of cholesterol causes plaque to accumulate inside the arteries, increasing the risk of a heart attack and stroke.

Reducing blood pressure may also boost heart health. Most individuals may do this by reducing their salt consumption to no more than 1,500 mg per day. Food makers add salt to many processed and quick meals, and a person who desires to decrease their blood pressure should avoid these goods.

Reduced cancer risk
A person may consume foods that contain antioxidants to help lessen their chance of getting cancer by protecting their cells from harm. The presence of free radicals in the body raises the risk of cancer, but antioxidants help eliminate them to lessen the incidence of this illness.

Many phytochemicals present in fruits, vegetables, nuts, and legumes work as antioxidants, including beta carotene, lycopene, and vitamins A, C, and E. According to the

National Cancer Institute, there are laboratory and animal studies that relate particular antioxidants to a lower risk of free radical damage linked to cancer. However, human studies are unclear and physicians warn against taking these dietary supplements without contacting them first.

Foods rich in antioxidants include:

- ☐ berries, such as blueberries and raspberries
- ☐ dark, leafy greens
- ☐ pumpkin with carrots
- ☐ nuts and seeds

Obesity may raise a person's chance of acquiring cancer and result in inferior results. Maintaining a modest weight may lessen these hazards. In a 2014 study, researchers showed that a diet high in fruits lowered the incidence of upper gastrointestinal tract malignancies.

They also discovered that a diet high in vegetables, fruits, and fiber lowers the risk of colorectal cancer, whereas a diet rich in fiber decreases the risk of liver cancer.

Better mood

Some data reveals a tight association between nutrition and mood. In 2016, researchers observed that meals with a high glycemic load may provoke higher feelings of sadness and tiredness in persons who have obesity but are otherwise healthy.

A diet with a high glycemic load comprises numerous refined carbohydrates, such as those found in soft drinks, cakes, white bread, and biscuits. Vegetables, whole fruit, and whole grains have a reduced glycemic load.

Recent studies have indicated that nutrition may impact blood glucose levels, immunological activity, and gut flora, which may affect a person's mood. The researchers also discovered that there may be a correlation between more nutritious diets, such as the Mediterranean diet, and greater mental health. Whereas, the reverse is true for diets with large quantities of red meat, processed, and high-fat meals.

It is vital to note that the researchers noted a demand for more study into the processes that connect diet and mental health. If a person believes they have signs of depression, discussing it with a doctor or mental health expert may help.

Improved gut health

The colon is filled with naturally occurring bacteria, which play key functions in metabolism and digestion. Certain kinds of bacteria also create vitamins K and B, which assist the colon. They may also help fight hazardous germs and viruses.

A diet rich in fiber may lower inflammation in the stomach. A diet rich in fiber vegetables, fruits, legumes, and whole grains may offer a mix of prebiotics and probiotics that assist healthy bacteria to grow in the colon.

These fermented foods are high in probiotics :
- yogurt
- kimchi
- sauerkraut
- miso
- kefir

Prebiotics may help relieve several digestive disorders, including irritable bowel syndrome (IBS) symptoms.

Improved memory

A nutritious diet may assist sustain cognitive and brain function. However, an additional definitive study is essential. A 2015 research discovered minerals and meals that protect against cognitive decline and dementia. The researchers found the following to be beneficial:

- vitamin D, C, and I
- omega-3 fatty acids
- flavonoids and polyphenols

- fish

Among other diets, the Mediterranean diet combines several of these components.

Weight loss

Maintaining a modest weight may help lower the risk of chronic health conditions. A person who has excess weight or obesity may be at risk of having several illnesses, including:

- coronary heart disease
- type 2 diabetes
- osteoarthritis
- stroke
- hypertension
- certain mental health conditions
- some malignancies

Many nutritious foods, including vegetables, fruits, and legumes, are fewer calories than most processed meals. A person can determine their calorie requirements using guidance from the Dietary Guidelines for Americans.

Maintaining a healthy diet can help a person stay within their daily limit without monitoring their calorie intake. In 2018, researchers found that following a diet rich in fiber and lean proteins resulted in weight loss without the need for monitoring calorie intake.

Diabetes management

A healthy diet may help a person with diabetes:

- manage their blood glucose levels
- keep their blood pressure and cholesterol within target ranges
- prevent or delay complications of diabetes
- maintain a moderate weight

It is crucial for persons with diabetes to minimize their consumption of meals containing added sugar and salt. They should also consider avoiding fried meals rich in saturated and trans fats.

Strong bones and teeth

A diet with appropriate calcium and magnesium is crucial for healthy bones and teeth. Keeping the bones healthy helps lessen the likelihood of bone disorders later in life, such as osteoporosis.

The following foods are high in calcium:
- dairy products
- kale
- broccoli
- scanned fish with bones

Food makers regularly fortify cereals, tofu, and plant-based milk with calcium.

Magnesium is plentiful in many foods, and some of the finest sources include:
- leafy green vegetables
- nuts
- seeds
- entire grains

Getting better sleep
A range of problems, including sleep apnea, may alter sleep patterns. Sleep apnea happens when a disorder persistently restricts the airways during sleep. Risk factors include obesity and consuming alcohol. Reducing alcohol and caffeine consumption may help a person get peaceful sleep, whether they have sleep apnea or not.

The health of the future generation
Children acquire most health-related behaviors from the people around them, and parents who model good diet and activity habits are likely to pass them on.

Eating at home may also help. In 2018, researchers discovered that youngsters who regularly ate meals with their family consumed more vegetables and less sugary items than their classmates, who ate at home less often.

There are dozens of minor methods to enhance a person's diet, including:

- exchanging soft drinks for water or herbal tea
- ensuring each meal includes some fresh produce
- choosing healthy grains instead than processed carbs
- ingesting entire fruits instead of liquids
- avoiding red and processed meats, which are heavy in salt and may raise the risk of colon cancer
- consuming extra lean protein, which individuals may obtain in eggs, tofu, salmon, and nuts

A person may also benefit from taking a cooking lesson and learning how to integrate more veggies into their meals.

Healthy eating offers several advantages, such as lowering the risk of heart disease, stroke, obesity, and type 2 diabetes. A person may also increase their mood and acquire more energy by keeping a balanced diet.

Chapter 2

With the stress of the COVID-19 epidemic weighing on individuals over the past year, it's more critical than ever to push for mental health services and daily routines that promote physical, mental, and emotional well-being. Even without a pandemic, Americans are concerned. About 33 percent of adults report experiencing high stress, and up to 73 percent indicate that stress damages their mental health.

Rest is crucial for better mental health, higher focus and memory, a stronger immune system, lower stress, improved mood, and even a better metabolism.

Importance of relaxation, rest, and sleep
So many Americans are mired in the grind of jobs, family duties, and chronic stress. Often, we only allow ourselves to genuinely relax during vacations. However, it's extremely vital to prioritize appropriate rest and quality sleep in

your daily life. Rest and sleep are two separate things, yet both are equally crucial to your mental, emotional and physical health. Plus, prioritizing rest might enhance your quality of sleep.

Rest may be difficult to describe since it might appear different for everyone. Rest is any activity intended at enhancing physical or mental well-being. It might be active, such as going for a stroll outdoors, or passive, such as taking 10 minutes to sit down and breathe deeply. Regardless matter how you choose to relax, these everyday habits may help you recuperate and recharge from physical and mental strain. That's why improved rest is connected to better physical and mental health.

Sleep, on the other hand, is a body-mind state in which individuals experience sensory detachment from their surroundings. Sleep is a crucial function of the body and affects every system from our cognitive function to immunological health. Quality sleep may help us refresh, recuperate and replenish. It's vitally crucial to brain function, memory, attention, immunological health, and metabolism. Unlike rest, sleep is something your body cannot operate without. If you are sleep deprived, your body will drive you to sleep, no matter what you're in the midst of.

Best tips

If left untreated, long-term stress may cause chest discomfort, headaches, digestive disorders, anxiety, depression, changes in sexual desire, and difficulty concentrating. It may not seem like a huge problem to omit to relax in your routine. However, there are various advantages to daily rest:

- lowered stress and anxiety
- better mood
- decreased blood pressure
- chronic pain relief
- improved immunological health
- stronger cardiovascular system

So, how can you better prioritize rest? Find modest methods in which you may include rest into your routine. We make time every day to eat, send our kids to school, run errands, and go to work. Why should rest be any different? Start by selecting a relaxing method that works for you. This might be meditating, doing yoga, strolling outdoors, listening to music, reading a book, having a bath, or any combination of these activities. When setting out your daily schedule, establish a regular time to relax. For example, you may take a calming bath before bed, practice meditation each morning or go for a brief stroll during your lunch break at work.

In addition to daily rest, it's advised that people obtain seven to eight hours of sleep each night, but the quality is just as essential as quantity. Rapid eye movement (REM) sleep is the most restorative of the five sleep periods. At least one-quarter of your sleep should be spent in the REM period.

How can you guarantee that you receive adequate quality sleep each night? You can:

- Avoid coffee in the afternoon and evening.
- Stick to a steady sleep routine, even on the weekends.
- Set your thermostat between 60 and 70 degrees at night.
- Avoid sleeping throughout the day.
- At least one hour before night, switch screen time for a calming activity such as reading, evening yoga, or a relaxing bath.

Exercise is crucial, but avoid working out late in the day, if possible.

Experts say you should strive to sleep between seven and eight hours of shut-eye each night, but what does that truly accomplish for you?

1. Sleep Can Boost Your Immune System

When your body receives the sleep it needs, your immune cells and proteins get the rest they need to fight off anything that comes their way — like colds or the flu. And according to the well-rested sleep professionals over at the American Academy of Sleep Medicine, regular sleep may also make immunizations more effective, which is a bonus.

2. Sleeping Can Help Prevent Weight Gain

Racking up eight full hours of sleep isn't going to result in reducing the lbs. by itself, but it may aid your body from loading on the pounds. If you don't get enough sleep, your body creates ghrelin, a hormone that promotes hunger. Your body also suppresses the synthesis of leptin, a hormone that signals you you're full. Put them all together and that's one deadly combination for late-night nibbling. Plus, when you don't sleep enough you feel more agitated and don't have the stamina to fight off junk food cravings. We're fatigued just thinking about it.

3. Sleep Can Strengthen Your Heart

Not getting enough sleep may lead to heart health concerns including high blood pressure or heart attacks. That's because lack of sleep may lead your body to generate cortisol, a stress hormone that drives your heart to work harder. Just like your immune system, your heart requires rest to work strongly and correctly. Just another reason to "heart" sleep.

4. Better Sleep = Better Mood

There is some truth in the ancient proverb, "Getting up on the right side of the bed." It has nothing to do with which side of the bed you roll out of, yet sleeping may contribute to pleasant emotions. And frankly, it makes sense. If you sleep well, you wake up feeling refreshed. Being rested helps your energy levels rocket. When your energy is high, life's tiny obstacles won't upset you as much. When you're not bothered, you're not as furious. If you're not upset, you're pleased. So, go to bed early and everyone around you will thank you for it.

5. Sleeping Can Increase Productivity

You may believe you're wowing your employer by burning the midnight oil, but putting off a decent night's rest might be having an unpleasant impact at work or school. Sleep has been linked to greater focus and higher cognitive performance, both of which may help you be successful at work. But one sleepless night might leave you feeling stressed, making it more likely that you'll make errors that a cup of coffee won't be able to remedy. Speaking of coffee, the more fatigued you feel, the more likely you are to grab that afternoon cup. And although that may appear to remedy the afternoon crash issue you have, the additional coffee late in the day might set you up for another restless night. Talk about a counterproductive cycle.

6. Lack of Sleep Can Be Dangerous. Literally. According to research from the AAA Foundation for Traffic Safety, you're twice as likely to be in a vehicle accident when you're traveling on six to seven hours of sleep compared to if you get a full eight hours. Sleep fewer than five hours and your chances of a crash triple! That's because your response time slows down when your brain isn't rested.

7. Sleep Can Increase Exercise Performance
Someone examined the effects of sleep
deprivation on basketball players and guess what
they found? When they didn't sleep well, they
weren't very good basketball players. Well, sleep
impacts all forms of workout performance.
Under-the-covers rehabilitation helps with
hand-eye coordination, response time, and
muscular repair. Plus, depriving oneself of sleep
might have a bad influence on strength and
power.

8. Sleep Improves Memory
Even if sleep offers your body the relaxation it
needs, your mind is still hard at work. It's
digesting and solidifying your memories from
the day. If you don't get enough sleep, who
knows where those memories go? Or worse,
your mind could fabricate false memories.

Sleep is nice. And essential. Roy Kohler, MD,
who specializes in sleep medicine at SCL Health
in Montana, repeats what we know about the
advantages of sleep, citing studies that reveal

individuals who get less sleep tend to be bigger, eat more, have a higher BMI, and are more likely to be diabetes. "Consistent sleep of seven hours a night is what's advised for adults merely for daytime functioning—being on task, being aware for the day, and being able to focus and not be so cranky and fatigued throughout the day," adds Dr. Kohler.

Chapter 3

Healthy connections with your spouse and family members may enrich your life and help everyone feel good about themselves. They don't simply happen, however; strong relationships take time to create and require effort to maintain their health. The more positive effort you put into a relationship, the healthier it should be.

People in healthy relationships love and support one another. They aid each other practically as well as emotionally. They are there for each other in the good times and the terrible ones. Healthy partnerships are generally founded on:
- respect
- trust
- open communication
- equality
- both shared and individual interests understanding
- honesty

- care
- emotional support
- shared beliefs on finances, child rearing and other vital factors

People who have good relationships are more likely to feel happy with their life. They are less prone to experience physical and mental health issues. Healthy partnerships can:

- boost your feeling of value and belonging and make you feel less alone
- give you confidence
- support you to try out new things and discover more about yourself

People that are in a good relationship speak to each other often and listen to one other too. Misunderstandings sometimes arise, and it can lead to individuals becoming angered, wounded, or puzzled. It is better to be explicit about what you want to express. Making a serious effort to grasp what the other person is saying also helps. Double confirming that you have understood accurately might avert misunderstandings. Just because you love each other doesn't imply you will be able to communicate properly or know what the other is thinking.

To promote more open communication in your relationship:

- set aside time to communicate with each other, without interruptions
- put yourself in the other person's shoes
- do not depend on the other person to guess what is going on, or how you are feeling
- listen to each other, and make sure the other person knows you are listening to them
- let the other person complete what they are saying
- talk about things honestly and politely
- try not to be overly defensive
- keep cool and try not to attack

Communication is not simply talking; non-verbal communication — your posture, tone of voice, facial expressions — may inform the other person how you feel. Non-verbal communication might even undercut what you're saying if your actions don't match your words.

Building strong connections with partners, friends and family is excellent for you. It enhances your mood, your mental health, and your wellness. Maintaining them is vital. It requires time and dedication. No relationship is flawless, but it must offer you more satisfaction than worry. Here are some guidelines for a good relationship.

Be clear about what you want
Assertive communication helps communicate your argument more clearly than passive or hostile communication. It implies you communicate your position clearly and honestly while respecting the other person's point of view.

Try utilizing 'I' statements instead of accusatory 'you' comments. For example, say "I detest it when you don't clean up the dishes" rather than "You never assist me in the kitchen".

Say apology when you're wrong
This is incredibly essential as it helps mend relationship breakdowns that eventually occur.

Be affectionate and express gratitude
Relationships may become routine after a time. Make special time together and continue to demonstrate your devotion. Even simply cuddling on the sofa after work can display closeness.

Make the connection a priority
It may be challenging to combine relationships, jobs, family, and friends. You can assist achieve a work-life balance by establishing boundaries at work and learning to say no – this will guarantee you make time for your relationship.

Develop common interests
Finding interests you both like helps you to spend time together. This might be as easy as

joining a night class together or taking up a new activity.

Work on feeling good about yourself
Feeling good about yourself allows you to give the best to your relationships. Taking time to do what you enjoy can help. Healthy friendships maintain your happiness and self-esteem, so you must stay in touch with your friends when you are in a relationship. One of the warning signs of an unhealthy relationship is when you quit activities you used to enjoy because of your partner.

Find solutions that work for both of you
Conflict is a part of any relationship. You both must recognize and embrace your differences and commonalities. Finding solutions that work for both of you will demand compromise at various times.

Make planning for the future
By establishing plans for the future together, you both demonstrate you are in the relationship for the long haul.

Family time
Finding time together as a family might be tough, but there are numerous advantages to regularly enjoying family meals. Even one family dinner a week provides everyone an opportunity to catch up, interact and engage with one another.

It is natural to experience ups and downs in a relationship. It is also natural to have various views. Relationships, and individuals, evolve throughout time. Your partnership is not healthy if one person has more authority than another, or if that person is abusive or aggressive.

Chapter 4

Exercise is the magic remedy we've always had, but for too long we've failed to take our suggested dosage. Our health is now suffering as a result. This is no snake oil. Whatever your age, there's substantial scientific evidence that being physically active may help you enjoy a better and happier life.

People who exercise consistently have a decreased chance of getting various long-term (chronic) diseases, such as heart disease, type 2 diabetes, stroke, and certain malignancies. Research reveals that physical exercise may also increase self-esteem, mood, sleep quality, and vitality, as well as lowering your risk of stress, clinical depression, dementia, and Alzheimer's disease.

Health benefits
Given the overwhelming data, it seems evident that we should all be physically active. It's

necessary if you want to live a healthy and
satisfying life into old age.

It's medically proven that persons who practice
regular physical exercise have decreased risk of:

- coronary heart disease and stroke
- type 2 diabetes
- bowel cancer
- breast cancer in women
- early death
- osteoarthritis
- hip fracture
- falls (among older adults)
- depression
- dementia

To be healthy, the UK Chief Medical Officers'
Physical Exercise Guidelines, advises that
individuals should strive to be active every day
and aim to complete at least 150 minutes of
physical activity during a week, using a range of
activities.

For most individuals, the best approach to begin moving is to make movement part of daily life, like walking for health or cycling instead of using a vehicle to get about. However, the more you do, the better, and taking part in activities such as sports and exercise can make you even healthier.

For any form of movement to help your health, you need to be moving swiftly enough to elevate your heart rate, breathe quicker, and feel warmer. This degree of effort is considered moderate-intensity activity. If you're working at a moderate level you should still be able to converse but you won't be able to sing the lyrics to a song.

An activity where you have to work considerably harder is termed robust intensity exercise. There is strong evidence that vigorous exercise may deliver health advantages over and beyond those of moderate activity. You can tell when it's intense exercise because you're breathing hard and quickly, and your pulse rate has gone up quite a little. If you're working at this level, you won't be able to utter more than a few words without halting for a breath.

People are less active today, partially because technology has made our lives simpler. We drive vehicles or use public transit. Machines wash our clothing. We enjoy ourselves in front of a TV or computer screen. Fewer people are performing manual labor, and most of us have professions that entail minimal physical exertion. Work, domestic duties, shopping, and other important tasks are significantly less taxing than for past generations.

We walk around less and burn off less energy than individuals used to. Research reveals that many persons spend more than 7 hours a day sitting down, at work, on transit, or in their leisure time. People aged over 65 spend 10 hours or more per day sitting or laying down, making them the most sedentary age group.

Sedentary lifestyles

Inactivity is defined by the Department of Health and Social Care as a "silent killer". Evidence is developing that sedentary conduct, such as sitting or laying down for lengthy periods, is detrimental to your health. Not only should you aim to boost your activity levels, but you should also limit the amount of time you and your family spend sitting down.

Common instances of sedentary conduct include watching TV, using a computer, driving the automobile for short travels, and sitting down to read, converse or listen to music. This sort of activity is considered to raise your chance of acquiring several chronic illnesses, such as heart disease, stroke, and type 2 diabetes, as well as weight gain and obesity. Crucially, you may accomplish your weekly exercise objective but still, be in danger of poor health if you spend the rest of the time sitting or laying down.

A lot of studies have indicated that exercise improves depression. There are several opinions as to how exercise helps persons with depression:

- Exercise may prevent unpleasant thoughts or divert you from everyday troubles.
- Exercising with others gives a chance for enhanced social engagement.
- Increased exercise may enhance your mood and improve your sleep habits.
- Exercise may also modify the amounts of substances in your brain, such as serotonin, endorphins, and stress hormones.

To preserve health and lower your risk of health issues, health experts and researchers suggest a minimum of 30 minutes of moderate-intensity physical exercise on most, ideally all, days.

Doing any physical exercise is better than doing none. If you presently perform no physical exercise, start by doing some, and gradually work up to the suggested level. Be active on most, ideally all, days per week.

Accumulate 150 to 300 minutes (2 ½ to 5 hours) of moderate level physical activity or 75 to 150 minutes (1 ¼ to 2 ½ hours) of vigorous-intensity physical activity, or an equal mix of both moderate and vigorous activities, per week. Do muscular strengthening exercises on at least two days each week.

Increases in daily activity may come from simple adjustments made throughout your day, such as walking or cycling instead of driving the vehicle, getting off a tram, rail, or bus a stop early and walking the rest of the way, or taking the children to school.

It is a good idea to contact your doctor before beginning your physical activity program if:

- you are aged over 45 years
- physical exercise causes discomfort in your chest
- you regularly faint or have periods of extreme dizziness

- modest physical exercise makes you extremely breathless
- you are at a greater risk of heart disease
- you fear you could have heart disease or you have heart issues
- you are pregnant.

Pre-exercise screening is used to identify persons with medical disorders that may place them at a greater risk of developing a health concern during physical activity. It is a filter or 'safety net' to help determine whether the possible benefits of exercise exceed the hazards for you.

Chapter 5

No matter the state of a statue, they are carved from the same stone—-similar to people from heredity. Statues are intriguing, even the damaged and incomplete ones. Like a marble statue, you are a piece of art, but it is vital to remember that you are also a work in progress. And you, too, can chisel yourself into a better person by being productive.

Even if you don't have your stuff together, you can still enhance your life. Contrary to what you may assume, you don't need Gucci footwear to take a step in the right way. You can take that step barefoot. You don't have to start off being the greatest; you simply have to start. Picasso undoubtedly experimented with finger paints before producing masterpieces.

When you're productive, you may grow other elements of your life, including your IQ, relationships, health, creativity, and muscles. Do this, and your life will match the ones in movies. What is important about developing yourself is that you're giving yourself your primary priority.

Being productive doesn't simply raise your bank account; it enhances your pleasure. It's the chicken soup for any soul: It stitches a shattered heart, alleviates physical pain, and cuts away at boredom — all while developing your body and mind. Who knew blood, sweat and tears could form a recipe for happiness?

Being productive gives you purpose.
No of your views, you may go to sleep with a dream and wake up with a vision. Having a precise aim will help you skyrocket out of bed in the morning like the fireball you are. Keep your sight on the prize, and concentrate on it. When you do this, all of your big-picture concerns will merge. Your happiness level will grow.

Being productive keeps your mind busy.
An engaged mind is a happy mind. Being busy gives no time for negative thoughts. You're not

thinking about Dave while you're teaching yourself Photoshop.

Learning gives you a cause to live. It greases your gears. In other words, eat your sweets, but don't forget to take your vitamins. When it comes to productivity, balance is crucial.

Being productive may boost your quality of life.
When you wear your passion like perfume, others — even your employer! — will take notice. Being motivated is key to unlocking increases and promotions. People argue that money doesn't buy happiness. It doesn't, yet no one is immune to the pull of a nice existence. With a little additional money, you can upgrade from your spring mattress. You may purchase medication that you might have been going without.

If you are currently living comfortably, you may relocate to a nicer place or spend some time for peace of mind on vacation.

Being productive might enhance your mood.
Productivity translates to various things for
different individuals. For others, it means
marking off fantasy places from their bucket list.
For others, it's something like exercise.

The Anxiety and Depression Association for
America informs readers on its homepage that,
according to certain research, "regular exercise
works as well as medicine" for some individuals.
And if you establish that you can be mentally
tough in a gym, you know that you can do the
same at an office.

Other de-stressors, including coloring, have
grown popular as well. Psychologist Gloria
Martínez Ayala revealed to The Huffington Post
why coloring lowers stress. Businesses have
listened: On lower Broadway, the Strand
BookStore dedicates numerous tables to adult
coloring books.

So, whether you're lifting a weight or a crayon, you have the power to clear your mind and lift your spirit.

Being productive helps you evolve.
Being productive teaches you to continuously push yourself. And the more productive you are, the easier it is to evolve into a better self. And because things in motion tend to stay in motion, being productive can easily lead to creating better habits.

Your schedule itself isn't important; whether you're a night owl or a morning bird, you can still be productive. As long as you keep moving forward and improving yourself, growth can take place at any hour. Start pushing yourself so much that it feels wrong to stay still. Find a comfort zone in being uncomfortable.

Being productive motivates the people around you.
When you inspire yourself, you inspire others.

And when you post motivational quotes, you're helping other people feel motivated, too. Some may claim that encouraging quotes clutter their news feeds. I would think they're influential. Words establish touch with people's eyes and hearts.

Doing your small dance invites others to make motions. And when others watch you develop, it gives them hope that they can do the same. Be proud of the job that you accomplish, and know that you prepare the road for those who praise you. Your steps create footprints for others to follow.

Chapter 6

Healthy thinking does NOT imply positive thinking! No one can look at things favorably all the time. Sometimes horrible things happen, like being fired at work, having a dispute with a friend, or losing someone you love. It's acceptable and good to feel unhappy and have negative thoughts when these things happen.

Healthy thinking entails looking at the full situation—the good, the bad, and the neutral parts—and then arriving at a decision. In other words, healthy thinking is looking at life and the universe in a balanced manner, not through rose-colored glasses.

Did you realize that your ideas have a huge effect on your mental health? That's because what you tell yourself about a circumstance influences how you feel and what you do. Sometimes your assessment of a situation might become twisted and you only concentrate on the bad aspects—this is natural and expected. However, when you view circumstances too negatively, you could feel worse. You're also more inclined to react to the circumstance in ways that are detrimental in the long run. Fortunately, there are specialized coping skills that assist handle challenging ideas.

What are frequent thinking traps?
Everyone slips into imbalanced thought traps from time to time. You're more prone to distort your understanding of things when you feel unhappy, angry, nervous, depressed, or stressed. You're also more prone to thinking traps when you're not taking good care of yourself, including when you're not eating or sleeping properly. See if you can detect your thought traps in the list below.

Overgeneralizing
Thinking that a terrible circumstance is part of a permanent cycle of awful things that happen. People who overgeneralize typically use terms like "always" or "never."

' I wanted to go to the beach, but now it's pouring. This usually occurs to me! I never get to do enjoyable stuff!'

Black and white thinking
Seeing things as just right or wrong, nice or horrible, perfect or dreadful. People who think in black and white terms regard a tiny error as a major disaster.
' I intended to eat better, but I just had a slice of cake. This strategy is a terrible flop!'

Labeling
Saying only nasty things about yourself or other people.
' I made a mistake at work. I'm dumb! My employer informed me that I made a mistake. My employer is a nasty jerk!'

Mind reading
Jumping to assumptions about what people are thinking, without any proof.
'My buddy didn't stop to say hi. She must not like me very much.'

Fortune-telling
Predicting that something horrible will happen, without any proof.
'I've been studying hard, but I know that I'm going to flunk my exam tomorrow.'

Mental filter
Focusing primarily on the bad features of a situation and dismissing everything nice or pleasant.
'I met a lot of fantastic individuals during the party, but one man didn't speak to me. There must be something wrong with me.'

Emotional reasoning
Believing that terrible sensations or emotions mirror the circumstance.

Discounting the positives
Believing that good things that happen to you don't count.
'My buddy complimented me on the food I prepared, but she was simply being kind.'

'Should' statements
Telling yourself how you "should" or "must" behave.
'I should be able to manage this without becoming upset and sobbing!'

How can I break out of a thought trap?

Here are useful techniques to combat typical thought traps. Many individuals feel their attitude and confidence improve after working through these abilities.

Don't attempt to break out of a thought trap by only telling yourself to quit thinking that way. This doesn't allow you to look at the data and confront the thinking trap. When you attempt to push painful thoughts away, they are more likely to keep creeping back into your mind.

1. Try to differentiate your ideas from real happenings
Ask yourself the following questions when something terrible happens:

- What is the situation? What exactly happened? Only include facts that everyone would agree on.
- What are your thoughts? What are you telling yourself?
- What are your emotions? How do you feel?
- What are your behaviors? How are you reacting? What are you doing to cope?

2. Identify the thought traps
Take a look at the ideas you've mentioned. Are you employing any of the thought traps and sliding into skewed thinking patterns? It's normal to slip into more than one thinking trap.

3. Challenge the thought traps

The greatest method to overcome a thinking trap is to look at your ideas like a scientist and analyze the facts. Use the evidence you've acquired to confront your thinking traps. Here are various methods to achieve that:

Examine the evidence

Try to find evidence against the thought. If you make a mistake at work, you might automatically think, "I can't do anything right! I must be a lousy employee!" When this concept comes up, you could confront it by asking, "Is there any evidence to support this view? Is there any evidence to invalidate this thought?" You could soon notice that your supervisor has appreciated your work lately, which doesn't support the assumption that you're a lousy employee.

Double-standard

Ask yourself, "Would I condemn other people if they did the same thing? Am I being tougher on myself than I am on other people?" This is a

fantastic strategy for overcoming mental traps
that entail severe self-criticism.

Survey Method
Find out if other individuals you trust agree with
your opinions. For example, you could have
difficulties with one of your kids and assume,
"Good parents wouldn't have this type of issue."
To counter this concept, you may ask other
parents whether they've ever had any troubles
with their kids.

Conduct an experiment
Test your views in person. For example, if you
believe that your friends don't care about you,
phone a few buddies and make arrangements to
meet together. If you anticipate that they would
all say no, you may be pleasantly surprised to
find that they want to see you.

Aim for a balance in your ideas
Once you have worked through some obstacles,
attempt to conceive of a more balanced notion to
replace the old thinking traps.

Are all negative ideas harmful thinking traps?
No—there are occasions when negative beliefs
are realistic. It might still be beneficial to
discover other ways of looking at the
circumstance, however. Try to identify a
significant personal challenge in the issue. See if
you can uncover any prospects for personal
improvement or skills development.

Many individuals living with challenging
circumstances discover that their distressing
thoughts improve when they focus on other
coping skills, such as recognizing the primary
causes of stress in their life, problem-solving
problems that they can control, and getting
social support.